AWESOME AT 50: BODY REBOOT IN 6 WEEKS

QUICK & EASY WORKOUT PLAN PLUS 30-DAY ASIAN MEAL PLAN

I. NGEOW

Written and illustrated by I. Ngeow

First published in Great Britain in 2020 by Leopard Print

Copyright © 2020 by I. Ngeow

CONTENTS

INTRODUCTION

CONGRATULATIONS ON MAKING THE first step. You're taking responsibility for your own health and fitness. Beginning is 80% of your goal. Completing it is the other 20%. Somewhere in between is where you can see your goal.

I hope the reason you're reading this book is because you are interested in the transformative effects of health and fitness at 50 and beyond. You want to be slim and healthy. You want to change. If so, you're in for a wonderful surprise. It is never a better time and it is not too late. I was born half a century ago and still am improving and learning every day.

There is nothing to buy. Your equipment list consists of this book, your own bodyweight, your mind, your sports bra, mat and water bottle.

I am an ordinary suburban working mom. Inside this book are no gimmicks, drugs, gadgets, Photoshop or filters. The photos you see in this book are snapshots and have not been retouched. I am all real and proud to be the age and the woman that I am. It took me 50 years to be this awesome. I don't see the purpose of photographic tricks.

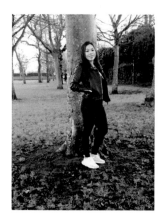

Your fitness will actually improve your hair and skin, increase your energy levels and enhance your emotional state. You won't believe the health benefits of health itself! People ask me how I achieve so much in a week, look after children, cook, clean, write, teach music and practice architecture. This is how. By being fit and healthy. If you are unwell or unhealthy you are bound to be inefficient at looking after your other interests, your family and least of all yourself.

If you are happy, your family will be happy and your doctor will be happy. It's a win-win, there are NO disadvantages of being fit. And it's free. I really cannot sell it to you more. You can look awesome at any age.

ESTABLISH YOUR AIMS AND OBJECTIVES

My aim was to lower my blood pressure first, as I have Stage One hypertension. If I lost weight or became slim, that would be a bonus. A 12-week program, with four sessions a week will be quite tough on your time commitment. Do that five times a week and you will see how much it has to cut into the other aspects of your working or family life.

I am not exactly lying down by the pool doing my nails all week. I also have a job to do and books to write. For a time-poor working mom, these programs were not ideal nor sustainable. In fairness at the time when I started doing 12-week programs, they really did the job, worked me hard and was what I needed and wanted. Ideally, we all should be exercising 5 days a week.

A few years passed and I had "done my time" doing other people's programs. I now have devised my own program for the time-poor working parent.

Before you get your exercise mat down and your leggings on, you need to ask yourself what is your fitness motivation and what are your goals? For example, mine was to lower my blood pressure. Now it is to have a flat tummy. Yours could be to lose weight or to be flexible or be fit and alert or have slim thighs. You could simply want to be more confident and relaxed. All of these goals are OK.

You can change your goals but you need to stick with one for as long as it takes. Most people give up on fitness and nutrition too quickly. Why? Because they never commit to one thing at a time. They want to do it all and they want it all, now. They want results in two days. There is no such thing.

We want to avoid such shocks to your body. One small step, giant leap etc. Always work methodically and put in your best effort each time. There are different exercises to realize different goals. Follow the rules and you will see guaranteed results.

HOW DO YOU KNOW IF YOU ARE FIT AND HEALTHY?

By the size of your waist. Forget everything else. The old common sense cliches are true: "keeping an eye on the waistline", "watching the middle-age spread," "losing an inch" etc.

"Keeping your waist circumference to less than half your height can help increase life expectancy for every person in the world," said Dr Margaret Ashwell[1], former science director of the British Nutrition Foundation. "The ratio was also better than just taking a waist measurement, as it took into account differing height between individuals and ethnic groups."

The team, who analyzed the health of some 300,000 people, found this ratio was a better predictor of high blood pressure, diabetes and cardiovascular events like heart attacks and strokes than body mass index.

Traditionally the Body Mass Index (BMI) has been used as an indicator of life expectancy and obesity. But BMI does not take into account the distribution of abdominal fat, around the heart, liver and kidneys, which has been found to be worse than that on the bottom and hips, in terms of heart disease and diabetes. BMI is calculated by taking one's mass in kilograms and dividing it by the square of one's height in metres.

Dr Ashwell said that waist-to-height ratio should be considered as a screening tool. Grab your tape measure now and do this simple test. For example:

If you are 6' (72") tall man, your waist measurement should be less than 36".

If you are a 5' 6" in (66") woman your waist measurement should be less than 33".

The second indicator of your fitness and health is wearing off-the-shelf clothes. For your height and clothes size, are your clothes pinching you at the waist?

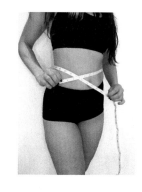

I am 5' 0" and I now have 26" waist after working on this aspect for many years, at my own rate. This correlates to 43%. Aim for 50% and if you fall under that, you're doing great, since clothes sizing go up in 2" increments.

I went from UK size 12 to 10 to 8. We all have our own body weight challenges and health issues. I have had 2 children and one Cesarean section. They cut my muscles and I will never have a completely flat belly. Just remember that nobody's perfect and never will be. So have no fear of trying to achieve it.

Watch the inches and the pounds will take care of themselves.

---

1. Adams, Stephen, Medical Correspondent, "Forget BMI, Just Measure Your Waist and Height", *The Daily Telegraph*, 12 May 2012

FREQUENTLY ASKED QUESTIONS

1. WILL I LOSE FAT AND SLIM DOWN?

You will. HIIT (see below) is how you burn fat. But the amount will depend on your age, previous training, genetics, how you're sleeping, what you're eating and how hard you exercise. The aim is to be healthier and leaner, and therefore any progress will be an improvement.

" Diet culture and the commonly held view that people in larger bodies are not as healthy as people in smaller bodies has a huge impact on, for example, self worth, self-confidence, access to medical care, of people in larger bodies.

People of all sizes can be healthy and eating good quality food and exercising regularly are key components of a healthy lifestyle."

---

2. WHAT IS HIIT?

High Intensity Interval Training is short bursts of intense exercise (also called cardio) followed by short rest periods. Repeat this pattern and that's it. HIIT burns calories for up to 18 hours afterwards even when you are not exercising such as when you are sleeping! Isn't that the best news? During your recovery, your body is working hard to repay the oxygen debt in your systems and restore itself to a resting stage. Your metabolic rate rises during the rest period so your body is burning more fat or more calories. During the intense part, work yourself hard as passible, so hard that you cannot speak. The harder you work the greater the oxygen debt therefore the more fat you will burn during the rest period.

3. ARE THESE EXERCISES FOR EVERYBODY?

Absolutely. Check first with your doctor if you have any health issues. The exercises are simple to follow. The first two sessions will be hard if you have never exercised before or have had a prolonged break. If it's too easy, work harder and if it's too hard, take a break or work less hard, but come back again and give it your best shot.

4. HOW DO I STAY MOTIVATED?

You can train with a friend or you can reward yourself after each session by giving yourself something pleasant (not food). If you do not want to do something, pay yourself. Put money in a jar and label the jar "shoe fund" or "holiday fund", for example. I believe in rewards. We reward children for good behaviour and it is how we train our minds and not just our bodies. Our body will start to obey. And in fact, after the first two weeks, guess what? You will start to see results and there is no greater motivation than results. Measure and weigh yourself before you start the plan. Also take photos of your front and side views in a swimsuit, underwear or bikini. Repeat in a month. Once you see yourself transformed, don't worry, you will be motivated.

5. WHAT SHOULD I DO BEFORE I START?

Book the time in, just as though you have meetings that you cannot miss. See the exercise journal section at the back of this book and fill the table in. Yes, you have very important meetings and it's with yourself. You are your own project. See it as beauty appointments or hospital treatments. Take it seriously. Don't leave it to chance or the table blank. You commit to it by writing it down. Keep track and count all your rounds. Each one takes you a step closer to being fit and lean.

6. DO I HAVE TO EAT WHAT'S ON THE MEAL PLAN?

You should but you don't have to stick to it religiously. It is an Asian-style portion control guide, and it's more like "trying on for size" only. Once you start eating less and cutting out the junk (sugar, high fat, high salt processed food, takeouts, instant supermarket meals, which means anything that comes in batter, a box or a bag), you won't feel like eating unhealthy food again. The meal plan is to only to help you avoid processed and/or junk food. With a regime or routine, it's easier not to be led astray or randomly eat because you have a plan that you will always be able to refer to. And then when you *do* go to restaurants or buy takeouts, you are much more aware that it is a total treat in itself and in fact you are probably a much better cook than the chef!

7. DO YOU HAVE ANY TIPS FOR EATING LESS?

Do not finish your children's or spouse's meals (which I have been known to do, since I am Asian). Save those for another mini meal, if you, like me, don't throw away food.

You'll also save money because you can stretch unfinished meals to another meal. No one ever told you that but it's absolutely common sense and true. Save money and slim down! It was how our forefathers survived from day to day in hard times, by splitting meals, eating half and saving the other half.

Drink water before eating. It will help you eat less because maybe you are actually thirsty. Always think before you put something in your mouth. Are you actually hungry or are you sad, bored, thirsty or all three? Build a relationship with food based on good habits.

Don't associate food with emotional needs. Think of the food you are eating rather than eating the food you are thinking of. You will NOT be hungry, because when you are hungry you WILL eat well.

It is eating badly that makes you hungry. Hence the vicious circle. The great news is that exercise curbs your appetite. Pair that with healthy eating and you have a winning combination.

More tips and expert advice will follow in the Nutrition Guide section of this book.

8. WHAT IF I'M TOO BUSY TO EXERCISE?

I am a busy working mom myself. That is why this plan has been designed. The shortest workout is 5 minutes and the longest 19 minutes long. This is a customized workout for the time-poor.

"Fit in fitness to be fit." - Ivy Ngeow

9. WHAT IF I DON'T LIKE EXERCISE?

You only don't like it because a) you ate the wrong things, b) you saw no difference and c) you gave up too soon. If you get all three right, it's a win-win. You will never dislike it again. In fact, you will love it so much you won't want to stop and you'll wonder why you didn't like it. Really. I know you don't believe me now, but 6 weeks from now, you'll laugh.

THE WORKOUT PLAN

THE PLAN IS BASED on 3 days a week of exercise. Allocate the three days by writing it in your exercise journal, calendar or timetable. For example, it could be Monday, Wednesday and Friday or Saturday, or Tuesday, Thursday and Saturday or Sunday. On the days "off" you should still carry out light activity for at least 30 continuous minutes of low impact exercise such as walking, swimming, cleaning, yoga, dance, or a sport such as tennis and badminton that gets you moving in an active or brisk way. The activity should not be passive or slow, such as shopping in a mall or "working". Shopping isn't really considered physical activity though some may argue that it is a competitive sport!

This 6-week plan is a high intensity interval training (HIIT) program which will both burn fat and add definition. Before you begin make sure you have

- an exercise mat
- T-shirt and shorts or leggings and a good sports bra
- a bottle of water
- an app timer on a phone or an old-fashioned timer. The

one I use is simply called Interval Timer. You can download this and program the timing in the settings. It is free and simple. I was using the app in seconds after I downloaded it.
- a towel (optional)

The first week will be an introduction or a warm-up. If you have exercised before it will feel very easy. If you have not exercised before, then it is a great way to start as they are short and sweet. They are designed to help you push yourself and do something new.

I am half-a-century year old working mom, a qualified writer, architect, makeup artist and musician. I am not a doctor, personal trainer or dietician. But I know what works on me, and it's being consistent with the program and the nutrition. That's why with the help of Joe Martinek of Jersey Joe Fitness in New Jersey, USA, I have come up with this customized body reboot workout plan for the time-poor. Joe Martinek is a NASM-certified ex-professional athlete and former New York Giants Football player. See www. JerseyJoeFitness.com and YouTube Channel JerseyJoe Fitness.

Joe says:

"To build muscle the idea is low reps, heavy weight, but to tone your body you want to do a lot of reps to help burn fat. I started each workout with base lift (working your bigger muscle of that muscle group) then supplemental exercises utilizing the surrounding muscles.

When you are building anything you need a good, strong base. You cannot build a concrete house on top of a wooden base. You will notice I gave you exercises with a lot of reps, that is to get your muscles used to lifting this much and build endurance. Also, as I said earlier it helps burn fat.

Before every workout make sure that you warm-up properly. The first set of the first exercise is somewhat of a warm up set. But before you start working out each day, you should work the muscles you are training that day. For upper body days I suggest doing some front, side raises along with push-ups."

Refer to the illustrations which explain the exercises but once you have learned them you will not need to check the diagrams again. You need very little space. You can do these exercises in your bedroom at home, a hotel room, a park, a poolside, anywhere. Just take this book with you.

If you're ready, let's begin.

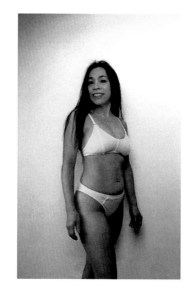

WEEK ONE

DAY 1

TOTAL: 5 minutes
    5 rounds
    20 second high knees running
    20 second body weight squats
    20 second burpees

DAY 2

Total: 4.2 minutes
    Front plank
    10 seconds | 20 second rest
    10 seconds | 20 second rest
    10 seconds | 20 second rest
    10 seconds | 20 second rest
    20 seconds | 20 second rest
    20 seconds | 20 second rest
    10 seconds | 20 second rest

10 seconds | 20 second rest
10 seconds | Finish

DAY 3

Total: 18 minutes
1 minute each exercise / 1 minute rest after each exercise
High knees running
Jumping jacks
Squats
Side leg raises (1 leg then other at half time)
Toe tap jumps
Lunge kicks (1 leg then other at half time)
Plank leg raises (alternating)
Mountain climbers
Plank jacks

WEEK TWO

DAY 1

TOTAL: 6 minutes
    Abs
    3 rounds
    1 minute rest between rounds
    15 second crunches
    15 second reverse crunches
    15 second air bike crunches (ab bikes)
    15 second flutter kicks

DAY 2

Total: 11.3 minutes
    5 rounds
    High knees running
    30 seconds | 15 second rest
    30 seconds | 60 second rest

DAY 3

Total: 10 minutes
    5 rounds
    1 minute rest between rounds
    20 second half jacks
    20 second side to side jumps
    20 second raised arm circles

WEEK THREE

DAY 1

TOTAL: 6 minutes
    Abs
    3 rounds
    1 minute rest between rounds
    20 second flutter kicks
    20 second sit-ups
    20 second sitting twists

DAY 2

Total: 10 minutes
    5 rounds
    1 minute rest between rounds
    15 second mountain climbers
    15 second plank leg raises
    15 second plank arm raises
    15 second plank jacks

DAY 3

Total: 11.3 minutes
    5 rounds
    Half Jacks
    30 seconds | 15 seconds rest
    30 seconds | 60 seconds rest

WEEK FOUR

DAY 1

TOTAL: 10 minutes
>   5 rounds
>   1 minute rest between rounds
>   15 second high knees
>   15 second side leg raises, alternating
>   15 second half jacks
>   15 second lunge step-ups, alternating

DAY 2

Total: 5.3 minutes
>   Abs
>   Move from one plank to the next with no rest in between
>   2 minute rest in-between rounds
>   2 rounds
>   30 second elbow plank
>   30 second plank

20 second raised leg plank (10 sec each leg)
10 second plank
10 second elbow plank

DAY 3

Total: 11.3 minutes
  Mountain Climbers
  5 Rounds
  30 Seconds | 15 Second rest
  30 Seconds | 60 Second rest

WEEK FIVE

DAY 1

TOTAL: 22 minutes
Elbow Plank
3 Rounds - 1 minute rest in between rounds
10 Seconds | 20 Second rest
20 Seconds | 20 Second rest
20 Seconds | 20 Second rest
30 Seconds | 40 Second rest
60 Seconds | 60 Second rest
20 Seconds | 40 Second rest
20 Seconds | 20 Second rest
10 Seconds | 20 Second rest
10 Seconds | Done

DAY 2

Total: 19 minutes
10 rounds - 1 minute rest between rounds

15 seconds elbow plank leg raises
15 seconds elbow plank jacks
15 seconds high plank arm raises
15 seconds high plank jump-ins

DAY 3

Total: 19 minutes
10 rounds
1 minute rest between rounds
30 second half jacks
20 second high knees
10 second mountain climbers

WEEK SIX

DAY 1

Total: 7 minutes
    Plank
    3 rounds
    1 minute rest between rounds
    30 second plank
    10 second push-up plank
    20 second plank
    20 second one leg plank (10 sec each leg)
    10 second one leg push-up (5 sec each leg)

DAY 2

Total: 19 minutes
    10 rounds
    1 minute rest between rounds
    20 second high knees
    20 second side leg raises

20 second mountain climbers

DAY 3

Total: 16.6 minutes
    Half jack floor taps
    10 rounds
    30 seconds | 10 Seconds rest
    30 seconds | 30 Seconds rest

NUTRITION GUIDE

DREAM (Don't Repeatedly Eat As Much) is an acronym I invented. DREAM is the natural, simple and sensible way to eat your way to great health, and the way it was always meant to be.

In this plan, you will consistently eat 3 meals and 2-3 snacks in between. Do not skip any meals or snacks. Ban any fads or diets or you will be tempted to overeat afterwards. Build good habits which will last a lifetime. In DREAM, you can forget about weighing or calorie counting, which is great news for the time-poor like myself.

You can eat whatever you want within reason, and you will still stay slim. "Within reason" means the amount that you eat should be proportional to you. We were born to feed ourselves with our own hands. Therefore, our hand size is all that is required to measure what we put in our mouths.

The guideline works like this:

- your protein in each meal should be fist-sized,
- carbs palm-sized, and
- vegetables or salad the size of two fists.

A cup size is roughly a fist. However, we all have different sized fists! So please adjust accordingly to your own anatomy.

According to Joe, and you may not like this (at first), you would have to cut out all salt and sugar. There is no need to add any of these to any meal.

"The hard part about attaining the physique you want is consistency, the even harder part is staring at a chocolate cake and saying no. Now I will give you some bad news before I give you good news. The bad news is YOU MUST CUT OUT ALL SALT AND SUGAR, no exceptions (meaning do not add excess salt or sugar to your meals, natural sugar is fine). Salt hold in water weight that makes you look and feel bloated and sugar helps store fat.

The good news, you do not have to eat salads for every meal.

The key to healthy living and complementing your workouts is healthy, PROPORTIONAL eating. So I just gave you bad news, some good news, now I am going to blow your mind.... you lose more weight the more you eat.

Now before you go crazy you need to listen, the science behind this is every time you eat your metabolism gets going. The faster your metabolism is the more calories you lose."

Occasionally you can eat whatever you like, greasy and/or sugary food. All these are part of our lifestyle and to cut them out completely would be much worse for your emotional well-being than to occasionally indulge and satisfy our desire for them. After that we may forget about them and get back on track. Food is not your enemy or your reward. It is enjoyable fuel. Always have a positive attitude towards eating.

Here are some good habits to make and some not too good ones to break, starting with regularizing your eating:

"You should target eating something every 2-3 hours, with doing this your metabolism stays active all day and you continue to lose weight even as you eat! Seems too good to be true right? The hard part is WHAT you are eating every 2-3 hours. Below I will lay out healthy snacks for you to eat but again it's all about proportions.

Stop yourself gradually from poor eating. Don't be too harsh as it has taken you years to form the bad habits so you need time to correct them. For example:

"If you are used to going to McDonalds every 4 days and get 3 dollar menu burgers every time you go, the next time you go start with 2 burgers (maybe not the greatest example but you know what I am trying to say!) The point is you do not have to drastically change your life, with my hints and tips you can eat tasty and still look damn good.

Nutrition will only get you so far without working out and working out every day will only get you so far if you eat ice cream every night. They both need to be in sync and working together."

Results come so quickly and within the first week, you will surprise yourself and may even treat yourself.

"I promise you the first week you collaborate your working out with your eating you will feel the best you have ever felt in your life. That's a Jersey Joe guarantee! If you thought staying consistent with your workout schedule was hard, your eating schedule is 10X harder, but not impossible. It makes it EVEN MORE difficult to stay on track when I tell you it's ok to have cheat days, yes have a candy bar, go get that fast food, as long as this is a once in a while occurrence (a reward for good behavior) there is nothing wrong with it."

Keep some variety. Eating healthy is not boring and neither is working out. Both are challenging physically and mentally. It is a sign of human intelligence to constantly evolve, maintain and motivate ourselves.

"The reason why you cannot keep doing the same workouts every week is because your body gets complacent, it is human nature. Think of this scenario; if you do the same exact thing every single day, you obviously get pretty good at whatever you are doing. After 2 years of doing the same thing, every day, you have mastered this skill, is there a reason for you to work hard at it anymore?

You get complacent and stop working hard and stop getting better. Same concept with working out and eating, you need to change things up and keep your body guessing. Keep challenging yourself to get better, keep trying to do something you have never done before. *Doing the same things over and over again and expecting a different result is the definition of insanity.*"

To summarize:

- *cut out the excess sugar and salt from your diet. You will see an IMMEDIATE body change.*
- *portion your meals out (have your big three meals of the day but in-between eat a healthy snack. Almonds are a*

healthy snack but 1 o handful of almonds do more harm than good,

- *cut out the junk food as snacks,*
- *find a healthy snack you can enjoy that gets rid of the junk food craving and remember to*
- *keep up with your workouts.*

7 TOP HEALTHY EATING TIPS

Joe's tips below will help you make good decisions today.

"Below are bullet points of tips on how to effectively eat healthy, knowledge is power and now you have the power to make good decisions.

• The feeling of your stomach "growling" is because your body is lacking fat to pick from. To stop this and get rid of your hunger for a brief time period, eat cheese. Cheese has the type of fats your stomach is looking for and eating a stick of string cheese is better than that bag of chips.

• Water intake is very important. Athletes are known to drink a gallon of water a day. Now for everyone that is not easy but I recommend always having a water bottle you can refill to keep with you throughout the day. Drinking water keeps your brain hydrated and makes you feel good. If you need that sugar taste (especially in the beginning) dilute your sugar drink (apple juice, lemonade, Gatorade, etc). Fill your glass a quarter the way of your juice and the rest of water. Obviously, the less juice you drink the better.

• A bottle of water after you wake up helps cleanse your stomach and makes it easier for your stomach to digest useful nutrients throughout the day.

• **Eat 80 percent of your diet in whole and minimally processed foods that you like**. "Whole" foods are ones that look like what they started out as: meat, fish, eggs, milk, nuts, seeds, fruits, vegetables, potatoes, and beans. One exception: Protein powders are highly processed, but they're still a great way to consume the protein you need to make the plan work.

• Eating protein in the morning there is a greater chance your muscles will absorb it.

• If the food doesn't have an ingredient list, it's a safe bet. Steak, apples, quinoa, eggplant, salmon—they're all single-ingredient foods. With packaged foods, each additional ingredient signals an extra step in processing, which may have stripped away some of the good stuff. And often, to make up for lost flavor, food manufacturers pump processed foods with sugar and fat. These foods also tend to be higher in calories.

• Eating peanut butter before bed is a good snack before you go to sleep. It takes your body a longer amount of time to breakdown peanut butter than most foods and you most likely won't wake up craving food. Because if you make a PB&J sandwich the sugar in jelly may make it difficult to fall asleep. Fun fact: body builders used to wake up in the middle of the night to eat, the thought process was would you ever go 8 hours during the day without eating? So why do it at night?"

In general and ideally these are the kind of foods that we will be eating in our meal plan:

- Meat and other protein-rich foods, including eggs and protein powder.
- Fat-rich foods, such as nuts and seeds, oil used for cooking or salad dressing, butter (and nut butters), olives, and avocados.
- Fibrous vegetables, including just about anything your mother said you had to eat if you wanted dessert.

- Starchy foods, such as grains (bread, cereal, pasta), legumes (beans and peas), and tubers (potatoes and other root vegetables).
- Milk and other dairy products, which includes all varieties of cheese, yogurt, and, yes, even chocolate milk.
- Fruits, fresh or dried.

7-DAY "MOCK" NUTRITION PLAN

You can use this as a template for your own life.:

MONDAY

Breakfast
3 scrambled eggs
1 large grapefruit
Snack
25 almonds
Lunch
Turkey wholewheat wrap
1 apple
Snack
1 piece of string cheese
Dinner
Spicy chicken and wholewheat pasta
Side salad and 2 tbsp olive oil/vinegar dressing

TUESDAY

Breakfast
2 tbsp of peanut butter with 1 piece of toast
1 banana
Snack
2 small boxes of raisins

Lunch

Leftovers

Snack

0% fat Greek yogurt

Dinner

Miso salmon

2 cups of broccoli

WEDNESDAY

Breakfast

Lean eggs and ham

1 large grapefruit

Snack

25 almonds

Lunch

Black bean and cheese burrito

1 apple

Snack

1 piece of string cheese

Dinner

Veggie Burger and bun

Salad with 4 Tbsp olive oil/vinegar dressing

1 serving of sweet potato fries

THURSDAY

Breakfast

Berry wafflewich

0% fat Greek yogurt

Snack

15 snap peas

2 Tbsp of hummus

Lunch

Sandwich

1 apple

Snack

1 banana

1 piece of string cheese

Dinner

Steamed Snapper with Pesto

1 cup of brown rice

2 cups of broccoli

FRIDAY

Breakfast

0% fat Greek yogurt

1 large grapefruit

Snack

Granola bar

Lunch

Salad

25 almonds

Snack

20-30 baby carrots

4 Tbsp of hummus

Dinner

Chicken Spinach Parm

1 cup of brown rice

2 cups of snow peas

SATURDAY

Breakfast

Loaded Vegetable Omelet

1 banana

Snack

1 piece of string cheese

Lunch

Turkey Wholewheat Wrap

1 apple

Snack

10 cherry tomatoes

2 Tbsp of hummus

Dinner

Quick Lemon Chicken with Rice

2 cups of broccoli

Snack

Sugar-Free ice-cream

SUNDAY

Breakfast

Loaded Vegetable Omelet

1 banana

Snack

15 baby carrots

2 Tbsp of hummus

Lunch

Eat Out

Snack

0% fat Greek yogurt

Dinner

Penne with Chicken Marengo

2 cups of broccoli

You do not have to follow the meal plan exactly, as mentioned in the FAQs. The idea is to replace it with a similar item in both portion and nutrition:

"Now, the goal is to give you enough information to make smart eating choices. So do not go replacing green beans with a McDonalds burger. If it says to have spinach but you do not have spinach or do not feel like spinach, then replace it with a vegetable you have/like."

A final word about portion size:

"Also, you will see I put things like "25 almonds", "30 baby carrots" do you have to eat exactly 25 almonds? No! Just do not eat 100. All about portion control. Same goes with those snacks, if you do not have access to them, replace them with something healthy to get you between meals."

Don't worry, you can cheat! Your body is clever and so are you.

"I have put in "cheat meals" in the plan because it is good to have them! Sometimes your body just needs to reset and eat something greasy. Because let's be honest, going 30 straight days eating perfectly healthy is close to impossible for 90% of us so a well-deserved break is good. But do not let that cheat meal carry over into other meals."

---

20 HEALTHY SNACK IDEAS
FOR YOUR MEAL PLAN

IN YOUR 30-DAY MEAL PLAN, you will see that you will need two to three snacks a day. They should be high fiber, high protein, low sugar and low fat. Don't skip your snacks but feel free instead to replace any of the snack items with the following list.

Each of these snacks are under 100 calories. You will see a few mentions of string cheese. This is mozzarella in a stick form which makes it a convenient, portable snack. One stick of part-skim string cheese has 80 calories and 8 grams of protein, plus a dose of calcium without the high saturated fat content of other cheeses.

If snacking is a mindless habit to counteract slight boredom and hunger, don't make the mistake of reaching for biscuits, bags of chips, salted fried nuts or prawn crackers which are high fat, high sugar, high carb and high sodium snacks. The sugar rush comedown is exhausting and will cause you to reach for more junk food to perk you up again. Instead, always prepare snacks ready in your bag or at home so that you will not be tempted to feast on unhealthy options, ruining the hard work you are putting into your workout.

- 1. A cup of blueberries.
- 2. A boiled egg
- 3. A handful of almonds
- 4. 1 tbsp homemade hummus
- 5. Chopped or cut vegetables eg bell pepper, carrots, cucumber or celery
- 6. A cup of strawberries
- 7. An orange
- 8. A pear
- 9. An apple
- 10. Half cup oatmeal
- 11. 2 cups baby carrots
- 12. One slice of toasted raisin bread
- 13. 30g high protein granola with 0% fat yogurt or skinny milk (skim)
- 14. Protein shake (a smoothie made with oat milk, 30g protein powder. Optional: a squeeze of honey and a tablespoon of berries)
- 15. Small skinny (skim) latte
- 16. 1 cup of melon
- 17. 1 banana
- 18. 0% fat yogurt
- 19. 2 cups air-popped popcorn
- 20. Half cup cottage cheese or tofu

30-DAY ASIAN STYLE MEAL PLAN

DAY 1

Breakfast

4 boiled eggs

1 large grapefruit

Protein shake

Snack

25 almonds

Lunch

Shrimp and quinoa lettuce wraps

1 cup of salad with 2 tbsp oil/vinegar dressing

Protein bar

1 apple

Snack

1 piece of string cheese[1]

Dinner

Chicken curry w/ 1 cup of brown rice

Half cup of vegetables

DAY 2

Breakfast
2 tbsp of peanut butter with 1 piece of toast
1 banana
Protein bar
Snack
2 small boxes of raisins
Lunch
Leftover chicken curry
1 cup salad
wholewheat pitta or naan bread
Snack
0% fat Greek yogurt
Shake
Dinner
Char siew grilled pork chops
1 cup of brown rice
1 cup of cucumber

DAY 3

Breakfast
4 scrambled eggs with ham or cheese
1 large grapefruit
Snack
25 almonds
Lunch
Udon noodles with leftover grilled pork chops

1 cup spinach

1 apple

Snack

2 pieces of string cheese

Dinner

Eggplant and okra (or sugar snap peas) sambal

1 cup of salad with walnut oil dressing

Brown basmati pilau rice

DAY 4

Breakfast

3 high protein low carb waffles w/ ¼ dsp syrup

0% fat Greek yogurt

Snack

1 cup snap peas

4 Tbsp of hummus

Lunch

Leftover eggplant and okra sambal curry

Half cup sugar snap peas

1 wholewheat naan bread or pitta bread

1 apple

Snack

1 banana

1 piece of string cheese

Shake

Dinner

2 cups of shrimp, Chinese cabbage and carrots

1 cup of quinoa

2 cups of spinach

DAY 5

Breakfast
2 tbsp of peanut butter in brown toasted sandwich
0% fat Greek yogurt
1 large grapefruit
Snack
1 pear
Lunch
Leftover shrimp, cabbage and carrots
1 cup of salad
25 almonds
Protein shake
Snack
30 baby carrots
1 boiled egg
Dinner
1 cup fish curry
1 cup of spinach
1 cup of brown rice
2 cups of green beans

DAY 6

Breakfast
4 egg-loaded vegetable omelet
1 banana
Snack

1 piece of string cheese

Shake

Lunch

Fish curry leftovers with salad

Protein Bar

1 apple

Snack

10 cherry tomatoes

2 tbsp of hummus

Dinner

Eat out

Dessert

Sugar-free ice cream

DAY 7

Breakfast

Oatmeal

1 banana

Snack

15 baby carrots

2 Tbsp of hummus

Lunch

Eat out

Snack

0% fat Greek yogurt

Protein shake

Dinner

2 cups wholewheat penne with chopped chicken in pesto 2 cups of
spinach

DAY 8

Breakfast
3 Scrambled Eggs
1 large grapefruit
Snack
25 almonds
Shake
Lunch
Leftover penne with chopped chicken in pesto
2 cups of spinach
Snack
1 piece of string cheese
0% fat Greek yogurt
Protein bar
Dinner
Ground Beef Thai style Lettuce Wraps
1 cup of brown rice
2 cups of snow peas
Snack
Air-popped popcorn

DAY 9

Breakfast
4 egg-loaded vegetable omelet
1 banana
Snack

2 piece of string cheese
0% fat Greek yogurt
Protein shake
Lunch
Leftover ground beef with chilli dressing and salad
1 apple
Protein bar
Snack
10 cherry tomatoes
Shake
Dinner
2 cups of tofu curry
2 cups of broccoli
1 cup of egg fried rice (brown)

DAY 10

Breakfast
3 Scrambled Eggs
1 large grapefruit
Snack
0% fat Greek yogurt
25 almonds
Protein shake
Lunch
Leftover tofu curry
2 cups of spinach
1 cup of brown rice
Snack
1 banana

2 pieces of grilled tofu

Dinner

Veggie burger and wholemeal bun

2 cups of spinach

DAY 11

Breakfast

2 Tbsp of peanut butter with 1 piece of toast

1 banana

Protein shake

Snack

2 small boxes of raisins

Lunch

Eat out

1 apple

Shake

Snack

1 Protein Bar

25 almonds

Dinner

Steak

1 cup of quinoa

Salad with 4 tbsp oil, mustard, honey and lemon juice dressing

---

DAY 12

Breakfast

4 egg-loaded vegetable omelet
1 large grapefruit
Snack
0% fat Greek yogurt
1 banana
Shake
Lunch
Steak sandwich on a slice of brown bread toasted
1 cup of cucumber
1 apple
Protein bar
Snack
15 baby carrots
2 Tbsp of hummus and chilli dip
Dinner
Honey grilled salmon in soy sauce, ginger and wine
2 cups of spinach
1 cup of quinoa

DAY 13

Breakfast
4 poached eggs and ham
1 Large grapefruit
Snack
1 piece of string cheese
25 almonds
Lunch
Leftover grilled salmon and quinoa wrap
1 cup tomato salad
1 apple

Snack

15 steamed baby carrots

Protein shake

Dinner

1 cup of brown rice

1 cup of 5-spice roast duck

2 cups of green beans

15 steamed baby carrots

DAY 14

Breakfast

2 slices of French Toast

1 large grapefruit

Snack

2 small boxes of raisins

1 piece of string cheese

Lunch

Leftover roast duck in hoisin sauce wrap with 1 cup of salad

1 apple

Shake

Snack

15 baby carrots

2 Tbsp of hummus

Dinner

Steamed chicken in wine and ginger

1 cup of broccoli

1 cup of brown rice

DAY 15

Breakfast
Oatmeal
1 large grapefruit
Snack
Air-popped popcorn
Lunch
Mediterranean hummus wrap
1 cup salad
1 apple
Snack
0% fat Greek yogurt
Protein shake
Dinner
2 cups of wholewheat soba noodles with sesame
1 cup steamed fish
1 cup spinach
Snack
Sugar-free ice cream

DAY 16

Breakfast
4 egg-loaded vegetable omelet
1 large grapefruit
Snack
2 piece of string cheese
Shake
Lunch
Leftover wholewheat soba fish noodles with vegetables

1 apple
Protein bar
Snack
25 almonds
Protein shake
Dinner
Slow-cooked chicken and ginger macaroni soup dinner
1 cup broccoli mixed with peas
1 cup of quinoa

DAY **17**

Breakfast
2 tbsp peanut butter oatmeal
1 large grapefruit
Snack
1 piece of string cheese
Protein shake
Lunch
Leftover chicken macaroni, ginger and carrot soup
1 cup broccoli and peas
Snack
0% fat Greek yogurt
30 baby carrots
Dinner
Sliced beef in oyster sauce with red and green bell pepper
1 cup of brown rice
2 cups of spinach
Salad with 2 Tbsp olive oil/vinegar dressing

DAY **18**

Breakfast
4 eggs and ham
1 large grapefruit
Protein shake
Snack
0% fat Greek yogurt
1 banana
Lunch
Tuna open sandwich on 1 slice brown bread and salad
Snack
2 piece of string cheese
Dinner
Grilled chicken breast burger and bun
Salad with 4 tbsp olive oil/vinegar/garlic dressing
1 serving of sweet potato fries

DAY **19**

Breakfast
2 slices of French Toast
Snack
1 banana
2 small boxes of raisins
Lunch
Leftover grilled chicken with salad
1 apple
Shake
Snack
15 baby carrots

2 Tbsp of hummus

1 piece of string cheese

Dinner

Eat out

DAY **20**

Breakfast

2 Tbsp of peanut butter with 1 piece of whole-grain toast

1 large grapefruit

Snack

25 almonds

Lunch

Eat out

Snack

1 piece of string cheese

Shake

Dinner

Grilled salmon with black sesame seeds

2 cups of green beans

1 cup of brown rice

DAY **21**

Breakfast

4 egg-loaded vegetable omelet

1 banana

Snack

1 Protein Bar

Lunch

Leftover grilled salmon, green beans and rice

1 apple

Snack

2 small boxes of raisins

Dinner

Thai ground beef with chilli in lettuce wraps

1 cup of brown rice

2 cups of snow peas

DAY **22**

Breakfast

4 eggs and ham

1 grapefruit

Snack

1 protein bar

Shake

Lunch

Eat out

1 apple

Snack

2 small boxes of raisins

Dinner

2 cups of wholewheat noodles and ground beef

1 cup of monk's vegetables (mixed)

Salad with 4 tbsp olive oil/vinegar dressing

DAY **23**

Breakfast

4 egg-loaded vegetable omelet

1 large grapefruit

Snack

1 piece of string cheese

Protein shake

Lunch

Leftover wholewheat noodles with ground beef and mixed vegetables

1 apple

Snack

25 almonds

Shake

Dinner

Grilled char siew pork chop or turkey breast

1 cup of brown rice

1 cup of broccoli

DAY 24

Breakfast

3 high protein low carb waffles w/ ¼ dsp syrup

1 large grapefruit

Snack

0% fat Greek yogurt

15 steamed baby carrots

Lunch

Tuna or egg sandwich, no mayo

1 cup cucumber

1 apple

Shake

Snack

Protein shake
Dinner
Steak
2 cups of spinach
1/2 cup of brown rice
15 steamed baby carrots

DAY **25**

Breakfast
2 tbsp peanut butter oatmeal
1 large grapefruit
Snack
0% fat Greek yogurt
Protein shake
Lunch
Leftover steak
2 cups of spinach
Airfried or oven-baked potato wedges/chips
Snack
25 almonds
Dinner
Chicken curry
1 cup of spinach
1 cup of quinoa
2 cups of green beans
Snack
30 baby carrots

DAY **26**

Breakfast

4 egg-loaded vegetable omelet

1 large grapefruit

0% fat Greek yogurt

Snack

1 Protein Bar

Lunch

Leftover chicken curry with quinoa and spinach

Dinner

Veggie burger with or without bun

Salad with 2 tbsp oil, honey, mustard and lemon juice dressing

1 cup sweet potato fries (oven baked or airfried)

Snack

1 apple

DAY **27**

Breakfast

2 tbsp of peanut butter with 1 piece of whole-grain toast

1 large grapefruit

Protein shake

Snack

10 cherry tomatoes

2 Tbsp of hummus

Lunch

Mediterranean hummus wrap

Tabbouleh salad

Shake

Snack

0% fat Greek yogurt

25 almonds
Dinner
Eat out

DAY **28**

Breakfast
2 slices of French toast
1 large grapefruit
1 cup of cottage cheese or silken tofu (bean curd)
Snack
1 pear
Lunch
Eat out
Snack
Handful of walnuts
Dinner
Soy sauce and sesame chicken with 1 cup of brown rice or
wholewheat pasta/noodles
1 cup broccoli with peas
Dessert
Sugar-free ice cream or frozen yogurt

DAY **29**

Breakfast
4 egg-loaded vegetable omelet
1 large grapefruit
0% fat Greek yogurt

Snack
1 protein bar
Berries shake

Lunch
3-bean and tofu salad (edamame, yellow beans, red aduki beans, tofu
and green leaf)
1 apple

Snack
2 small boxes of raisins

Dinner
2 cups of brown rice with grilled fish
Half cup of quinoa
1 cup steamed pak choy

DAY **30**

Breakfast
Oatmeal
1 large grapefruit
0% fat Greek yogurt

Snack
25 almonds
Protein shake

Lunch
Asian Chicken Salad (dressing: soy sauce, garlic paste, sesame oil, red
chillies and honey)
1 apple

Snack
2 pieces of grilled tofu

Dinner

Lean ground beef, turkey or pork with wholewheat noodles
2 cups of spinach
1 cup of quinoa

---

1. String cheese is string mozzarella. Throughout the plan, you can substitute it with mozzarella pearls, vegan mozzarella or tofu. Do not mistake it for Cheestrings which is a kids' cheese snack.

EXERCISE JOURNAL

Jot down the week number, day and date. Count the rounds and mark them down as done.

#success !

Refer to the example for Week 1, Day 1, and print or simply fill in the blank one with your own records.

Example:

WEEK.	DAY.	DATE.	ROUNDS.	DONE.
W1	1. TUES	24 DEC 19	𝍸	✓
	2. THURS	26 DEC 19	|	✓
	3. SAT	28 DEC 19	|	✓

Actual journal:

WEEK.	DAY.	DATE.	ROUNDS.	DONE.
W1	1.			
	2.			
	3.			
W2	1.			
	2.			
	3.			
W3	1.			
	2.			
	3.			
W4	1.			
	2.			
	3.			
W5	1.			
	2.			
	3.			
W6	1.			
	2.			
	3.			

ILLUSTRATIONS

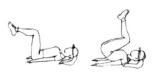

Reverse crunch.

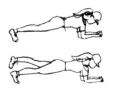

Plank leg raise.

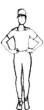

Side leg raise.

Crunches.

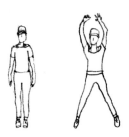

Jumping jacks.

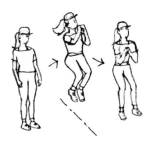

Side to side jumps.

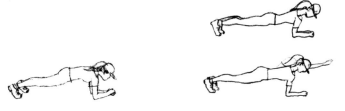

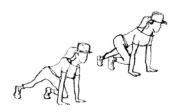

Plank.

Plank arm raise.

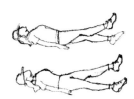

Mountain climbers.

Flutter kicks.

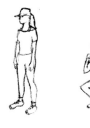

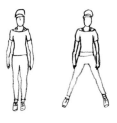

Squats.

Half jacks.

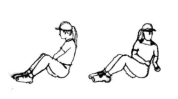

Sitting twists.

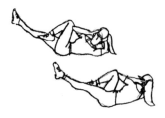

Ab bikes.

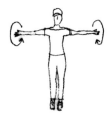

Raised arm circles.

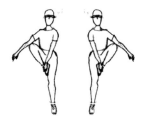

Toe tap jumps.

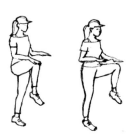

High knees running.

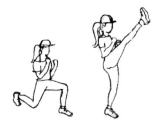

Lunge kicks.

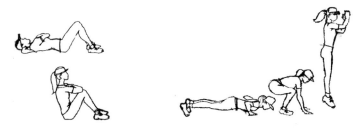

Sit-ups.

Burpees.

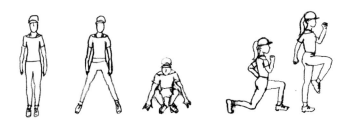

Half jack floor taps.

Lunge step-ups.

WANT MORE?

NOW THAT YOU'VE **completed your 6-week challenge, guess what?** Here's some great news for you. You can move on to specific abs workouts. How would you like to have a smaller waistline in just 2 weeks? **Take the challenge and flatten that curve with this gym-free, quick and easy workout guide and 14-day meal plan,** *Amazing at 50: 10-day Flat Tummy Challenge.* For the over-50s, or anyone who wants to watch the waistline and develop healthy eating habits. Read *Amazing at 50: 10-day Flat Tummy Challenge.*

Get organized with your routines. If you are trying to keep track of what you eat and how active you are so you can improve your diet and daily routines, then *Fitness and Meal Plan Journal: 12-Week Daily Workout and Food Planner Notebook* will be your friend and coach in your journey to becoming the healthier you. This no-nonsense, quick and easy-to-use organizer is available in a handy and portable 9" x 6" paperback format. Read *Fitness and Meal Plan Journal: 12-Week Daily Workout and Food Planner Notebook.*

BEFORE YOU GO

The book you are holding in your hand is the result of my dream to be an author. I hope you enjoyed it as much as I enjoyed writing it. I am slowly building my author brand, ranking and profile. As you probably suspected, it takes weeks, months or years to write a book. It exists through dedication, passion and love. Reviews help persuade others to give my books a shot. More readers will motivate me to write, which means more books. I love connecting with and hearing from you. I personally read each review you write. It gives me a sense of fulfilment and meaning— you read my book, I read your review. It will take *less than a minute* and can be *just a line* to say what you liked or didn't. If you could do me just this one favour and help me, I would be ever so grateful. Please leave me a review wherever you bought this book from. A big thank you. *Ivy*

"The longer I live the more beautiful life becomes."
- Frank Lloyd Wright

ABOUT THE AUTHOR

I. Ngeow was born and raised in Johor Bahru, Malaysia. A graduate of the Middlesex University Writing MA programme, Ivy won the 2005 Middlesex University Literary Press Prize out of almost 1500 entrants worldwide. Her debut *Cry of the Flying Rhino* (2017) won the 2016 International Proverse Prize.

A regular suburban London mum who likes books, wine and cake, Ivy has had a passion for creative writing since she was a child, winning her first competition at 16. She started writing non-fiction lifestyle books to help families or busy and tired people, like herself, to save time and money by cooking and keeping fit at home in modern, quick and easy ways. Her interests include impromptu virtuoso piano performances, health and fitness, beauty and sewing. You can find her here:

writengeow (www.writengeow.com)
Twitter (twitter.com/ivyngeow)
Facebook (facebook.com/ivyngeowwriter)
Instagram (www.instagram.com/ivyngeow)
Email: ivy_ngeow AT yahoo DOT com

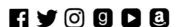

ALSO BY I. NGEOW

COOKBOOKS

30 Chinese Dinners: Healthy Easy Homemade Meals

Quick and Easy Party Treats: for special occasions

FITNESS

Fitness and Meal Plan Journal: 12-week daily workout and food planner notebook

Amazing at 50: 10-day Flat Tummy Challenge

Awesome at 50: Body Reboot in 6 weeks

DESIGN

Midcentury Modern: 15 Interior Design Ideas

ACKNOWLEDGMENTS

I WOULD LIKE TO thank Joe Martinek of Jersey Joe Fitness in New Jersey, USA, for helping me to put together this concise workout plan and meal plan and contributing to the guide. Dr Catherine Wall for feedback on the meal plan. My parents for giving me the genetics that I was born with. My family who taught me to love and to value life: firstly, I don't need a gym because they are my gym. Secondly, through looking after them and cooking easy meals from scratch, I became aware of the benefits of simplifying health. Thirdly, my daughter, 40 years my junior, whose love for ballet, music, baking and gymnastics inspired my interest in dance, fitness and healthy living when I was already nearly 50. Lastly, my friends and my Instagram and Twitter followers who have become friends. You've always been there for me, supported my artistic endeavors and my pursuit of a life more meaningful. May we all live a beautiful life.

To all of you, my special thanks.